# YOUR KNOWLEDGE HAS VALUE

AF166956

- We will publish your bachelor's and master's thesis, essays and papers

- Your own eBook and book - sold worldwide in all relevant shops

- Earn money with each sale

## Upload your text at www.GRIN.com and publish for free

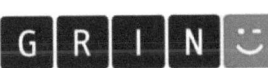

# Guarding Against Pertussis. The Efficacy and Advantages of the TdaP Vaccine

Hyacinthe Tuyubahe Praveen Kumar Vemuri

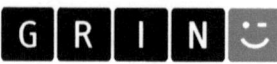

**Bibliographic information published by the German National Library:**

The German National Library lists this publication in the National Bibliography; detailed bibliographic data are available on the Internet at http://dnb.dnb.de.

ISBN: 9783346908599
This book is also available as an ebook.

© GRIN Publishing GmbH
Trappentreustraße 1
80339 München

Print and binding: Books on Demand GmbH, Norderstedt, Germany
Printed on acid-free paper from responsible sources.

The present work has been carefully prepared. Nevertheless, authors and publishers do not incur liability for the correctness of information, notes, links and advice as well as any printing errors.

GRIN web shop: https://www.grin.com/document/1351272

# Indigenous technology for purification of Vaccine components from *Bordetella pertussis*

# ABSTRACT

The increased risk of pertussis in adults have become an important public-health issue. This contagious disease spreads to infants who have lesser immunity resulting in their death. Increased death rate caused the inventions of vaccinations to prevent this disease. Concerns regarding the safety of whole-cell vaccines used for pertussis treatment lead to the development of acellular pertussis vaccines like TdaP vaccines. This combination vaccine is 71-85% effective in the treatment of adults suffering from diseases tetanus, diphtheria and pertussis. These vaccines have limited side effects when compared to whole-cell vaccines as they contain purified antigenic components of *Bordet Ella pertussis* (Pertussis toxin, Filamentous hemagglutinin and Pertactin) that are obtained by the purification techniques Tangential flow filtration, Column Chromatography and Dialysis. These components are then formulated for purified vaccine production.

## OBJECTIVE

To purify pertussis toxin, filamentous hemagglutinin and pertactin from Bordetella pertussis for development of the vaccine

# ABBREVATIONS

| | | |
|---|---|---|
| ACIP | - | Advisory common Immunization Practices |
| aP | – | Acellular pertussis |
| CDC | – | The Centers for Disease Control and Prevention |
| CV | – | Column Volume |
| DF | - | Diafiltration |
| DTaP | – | Diphtheria, Tetanus, Acellular Pertussis |
| DTP | - | Diphtheria Toxoid Pertussis |
| EUVAC | - | Electronic Discrete Variable Automaticic Computer |
| HA | – | Filamentous Hemagglutinin |
| HIC | – | Hydrophobic interaction Chromatography |
| HPLC | – | High Performance Liquid Chromatography |
| Hrs | - | Hours |
| Min | - | Minutes |
| mL | – | Milli liter |
| NA | - | Not Available |
| Nm | - | Nanometer |
| PCR | - | Polymer Chain Reaction |
| PFGE | - | Pulsed Field Gel Electrophoreosis |
| PRN | - | Pertactin |
| PT | – | Pertussis Toxin |
| RGD | - | Arginine, Glycine, and Aspartate |
| SNPex | - | Single nucleotide Primer extension |
| TdapP | – | Tetanus, Diphtheria, Acellular Pertussis |

| | | |
|---|---|---|
| TFF | – | Tangential Flow Filtration |
| UF | - | Ultrafiltration |
| US | - | United States |
| Vag | - | Vaginal |
| WBC | - | White Blood Cells |
| WHO | – | World Health Organization |
| wP | – | Whole-cell Pertussis |

# 1. Table of Contents

Editor's Note: Some figures were removed due to copyright issues.

# 2. INTRODUCTION

## 2.1 VACCINE:

Vaccine is a substance, which stimulates the production of antibodies and provides immunity against several diseases. It is prepared from the causative agent of the disease, its products or synthetic substitutes. In treatments, it is used to act as an antigen without inducing the disease. Vaccine provides active acquired immunity to a particular disease and it consists of an agent that resembles a disease-causing microorganism that is made from weakened or killed forms of the microbe, its toxin or one of its surface proteins. It protects people from serious and deadly diseases.(1,2)

### 2.1.1 HOW VACCINES ARE USED:

It is a type of medicine that trains body's immune system to fight a disease it has not metbefore. Vaccines are mainly used to prevent diseases. They are mostly given as an injection (needle). Some are given orally (mouth) or nasally (sprayed into the nose). (3,4)

### 2.1.2 VACCINATION:

The act of introducing vaccine into a body to provide immunity to a particular disease is termed as **vaccination. (5)**

## 2.2 BORDETELLA PERTUSSIS

### 2.2.1 ABOUT BORDETELLA PERTUSSIS:

*Bordet Ella pertussis*, gram-negative bacteria that is an encapsulated coccobacillus of the genus *Bordet Ella* causes the disease pertussis or whooping cough. It is an aerobic, pathogenic bacterium, which is motile and has a flagellum-like structure.(6)

### 2.2.2 CAUSE OF DISESASE THROGH BACTERIA:

This bacteria is transmitted through droplets released by the person having whooping cough. After entering into the host body the bacteria colonizes only on the ciliated cells of the respiratory mucosa and spreads rapidly. Eventually they release toxins like pertussis toxins (PT) and others that damage cilia andcauses airways to swell making that person difficult to breathe. The attachment of bacteria to the ciliated cells are facilitatd by proteins called as filamentous hemagglutinin (FHA) and pertactin (PRN). These three proteins are the antigenic components that are purified and used in making vaccines after detoxification.

### 2.2.3 TYPES OF PERTUSSIS VACCINE:

Pertussis is prevented using pertussis vaccines. These vaccines are of two types: whole-cell vaccines and acellular pertussis vaccines (acellular vaccines). Concerns regarding the safety of whole-cell vaccines prompted the development of acellular pertussis vaccines which does not have any adverse effects as it contains purified antigenic components of Bordet Ella pertussis. It is also called as DTaP(diphteria, tetanus and pertussis) vaccine and Tdap (tetanus, diphteria and pertussis) vaccine. DTaP is used for children and Tdap for adults. Tdap offers the best prevention and is marketedunderthe brand names ADACEL and Boostrix.

### 2.2.4 PURIFICATION OF VACCINE

Isolation of one or more proteins from a complex mixture like cells, tissues or whole organisms are done by a series of processes called protein purification. This process separates protein and non-protein parts of the mixture and thus the desired protein can be isolated. The characterization of structure, functions and interactions of the protein of interest can be done by protein purification. Chromatographic techniques (Cation exchange and anion-exchange chromatography, etc.), Tangential flow filtration and Dialysis are mainly used for protein purification. These methods are used tomake acellular pertussis vaccines from the bacteria *Bordet Ella pertussis* so that purified vaccines can be obtained.(7)

### 2.3 PERTACTIN (PRN)

#### 2.3.1ORIGIN OF PRN

In microbiology, pertactin (PRN) is a highly immunogenic virulence factor of *Bordetella pertussis*, the bacterium causes pertussis. Specifically it is an outer membrane protein promotes adhesion to tracheal epithelial cells.PRN is used to produce vaccine; it is one of the important component in producing acellular pertussis vaccine. (8)

#### 2.3.2 STRUCTURE OF PRN

In PRN, the large part of N-terminates was composed of beta-helix repeats(9). In this region the amount of protein was secreted by the C-terminal auto transporter. The N-terminal signal sequences promotes the secretion of PRN into the periplasm through the bacterial secretion system(Sec) and consequently,the translocation into the outer membrane where it is proteolytically cleaved.The loops in the right-handed beta-helix of the N-terminus that protrudes the outer of cell surface(region R1)contains sequence repeats Gly-Gly-Xaa-Xaa-pro and the RGD domain Arg-Gly-Asp.The RGD domains allows PRN to function as an adhesion and invasion,bindind into integirns and outer membrane of the cell.Another loops of extending beta-helix in region 2 (R2) which contains Pro-Gln-Pro (PQP) repeats towards the C-terminus.The protein's contribution to immunity is still premature.Reports suggest that R1 and R2 are immunogenic regions,however,recent studies regardindgentic variation of those region prove otherwise.(10)

## 2.4 FILAMENTOUS HEMAGGLUTION(FHA)

### 2.4.1 ABOUT FHA

The filamentous hemagglutininadhesin (FHA) is a large, filamentouspritein that serves as a dominant attachment factor adherence to host ciliated epithelial cells of the respiratory tracks ,called respiratory epithelium(11). It is associated with biofilm formation and possesses at least four binding domains which can bind in different cell receptorson the epithelial cell surface.One notable bacterium that produces filamentous heamagglutiumadhesin is *Bordetellapertussis*,which uses this protein asa virulence factor.(12)

### 2.4.2 NUCLEOTIDE SEQUCENCE OF FHA

Filamentous heamagglutlum is asurface- associated adherence protein of*Bordetollapertussis*,which is a component of some new acellular pertuissvaccines.The nucleotide sequence of open reading frame that encompasses the filamentous heamagglutium structural gene,fhaB,suggests that proteolytic processing is necessary to generate the mature 220-kDa filamentous heamagglutiumproduct.AnArg-Gly-Asp(RGD) tripeptide found within filamentous heamagglutinin that maybe involved in its adherence properties.Aninternal in-frame deletion fhaB,encompassing the RGD region,cause loss of B.Pertuiss-binding to ciliated eukrayticcells,confirming a potential role for this protein in host-cell binding and infection.

# 3. REVIEW OF LITERATURE

3.1 AIM OF REVIEW:

Bordet was awarded the 1919 Noble Prize in Physiology and Medicine at 1920 for his study in the field of antimicrobial immunology that contained extensive study of *Bordetella pertussis*, the causative agent of whooping cough (13).

3.2 MICROBIOLOGY OF BORDETELLA SPECIES:

Bordetella species comprised of 10 genetically distinct species comes under the family of Alcaligenaceae (2-3). *Bordetella pertussis* is a gram-negativebacterium, which grows optimally from the range 35 -37on either Bordet-Gengou or Regan-Lower agar. It is distinguished from other species of bordetella depending on their growth and biochemical characteristics (12, 13, 29-32). They also grow slowly on the synthetic and blood supplement media, which has appropriate growth factors like nicotinamide (3).

## 3.3 MECHANISMS OF PATHOGENESIS:

*Bordetella pertussis* a human-specific pathogen (55–58). The synchronized interaction of various virulence factors of *Bordetella pertussis* such as, pertussis toxin (PT), Adenylate cyclase toxin (AC), dermonecrotic toxin (DNT), and tracheal cytotoxic (TCT) results in pertussis. Many other factors have an impact on the virulence of *Bordetella pertussis* that include the surface structures like filamentous hemagglutinin (FHA), fimbriae (FIM), pertactin (PRN), the type III secretion system, lipopolysaccharide (LPS) and metabolic proteins (e.g.: BrkA,BapC).Other factors that influence the virulence of *Bordetella pertussis*incide surface structure , such as filamentous hemagglutinin (FHA),fimbriae (FIM),pertacin(PRN),the type 3 secretion system,and lipopolysaccharide (LPS) (59), and metabolic proteins e.g.,BrkA,BapC,andBatB(60-132).In B.pertuiss, the bvgAs genes positively control       expression       of       several       virulence       factors,including PT,AC,DNT,TcfA,FHA,pertactin,FIM,BrkA,BipA,BcfA,and Vag8.The BvgAS two – component signal transduction system of Bordetellapertuissis plays a pivotal role in pertussis pathogenicity (133,134).Bordetellapertuissispathogenisis is influenced by causes(e.g., temperature changes) that dictate virulence factor expression once inside the human host. During transmission from person to person, *Bordetella pertussis*moves fromlocal environmental temperatures to higher body temperatures which appear to influence regulation of the bvgAand bvgSgenes (135). In turn, the regulatory system encoded by bvgAand bvgScan be activated by temperature (as well as sulfate [SO4] and nicotinate) and regulates expression of virulence factors in *Bordetella pertussis*and Escherichia coli (136–138). The mechanisms of virulence of*Bordetella pertussis*consist of a cascade of events initiated by the adherence of bacteria via FHA and fimbriae to tracheal epithelium and lungs as an essential primary step (141, 142). Once adherence takes place, *Bordetella pertussis*cells multiply locally, resist host defense mechanisms (e.g., mucociliary clearance, antimicrobial peptides, and inflammatory cells), and cause local damage to the upper and lower respiratory tracts with systemic manifestations (143–145). The severity of the symptoms depends on several factors, including the patient's age, strength of the immune response, and extent of systemic bacterial dissemination. In infants, for whom disease is severe, bacteria descend from the upper to the lower respiratory tract and, via an unclear mechanism, produce necrotizing bronchitis, diffuse alveolar damage, intra-alveolar hemorrhage, fibrous edema, macrophage-rich alveolarinfiltrates, lymphangiectasia, neutrophilic bronchopneumonia, and fibrin thrombi (142, 143, 146). In more severe cases, these pathological events can lead to pulmonary hypertension, respiratory failure, and even death (142, 147, and 148). Pulmonary hypertension develops as an indirect effect of PT through induction of lymphocytosis (hyper leukocytosis), in which the total white blood cell (WBC) count can exceed 1 _ 105 cells/mm3.These extremely high WBC counts produce lymphocyte aggregations in the pulmonary vasculature that result in increased pulmonary vascular resistance (149–151). In infants with pertussis, the lymphoid system is also affected. Postmortem biopsies have shown cortical atrophy of the thymus gland, lymph depletion in lymph nodes, and white pulp depletion in spleen (152). In infantswho had encephalopathy secondary to *Bordetella pertussis*infection, brain biopsies showed cerebral hemorrhage and cortical atrophy (153,154). Although these pathological findings could result from the direct effect of *Bordetella pertussis*toxins on the brain, they are thought to result from hypoxia (145).

### 3.4 EPIDEMIOLOGY:

#### 3.4.1 Global burden of Pertussis

Pertussis is an endemic disease in developing and developed countries, with frequent outbreaks occurring sporadically at different places around the world. In 1999, Crow croft et al. estimated theglobal incidence of pertussis to be 48.5 million cases, with approximately295,000 deaths reported (155). In 2010, Black et al. reportedthat 16 million cases of pertussis occurred in 2008 worldwide,resulting in 195,000 deaths (156). A large number of deaths(83,580) were reported from Africa (156, 157). In 2013, an estimated 136,000 cases worldwide were reported (158, 159). There are several challenges in estimating the global pertussisdisease burden. First, many countries have limited surveillanceinfrastructure, which does not facilitate timely reporting of clinicallysuspected pertussis cases. Second, in developing countries,laboratory infrastructure to support routine pertussis testing is limited, and molecular diagnostic tests such as PCR are not uniformly available (160). Third, in areas with few trained healthprofessionals, inconsistent clinical identification of pertussis diseasemay hinder case reporting. The working group found that the evaluation of pertussis incidence is a complex task at the global and country levels. Estimating the burden of pertussis has been a major challenge due to several factors, including changes in surveillance and diagnostic methods over time, changes in national vaccine schedules for and compositions of diphtheria toxoid–tetanus toxoid–whole-cell pertussis (DTP) or diphtheria toxoid-tetanus toxoid-acellular pertussis (DTaP) vaccines, and changes in vaccine manufacturers (161).

#### 3.4.2 BURDEN OF PERTUSSIS IN INFANTS AND TODDLERS

In the vaccine era (from the 1940s to the present), pertussis epidemics have occurred in 3- to 4-year cycles that may have resulted from the cycling of population immunity (188, 189). In the United States, pertussis has become endemic and is currently considered the most common vaccine-preventable disease (190–195). Recent nationwide incidences of pertussis for children less than 6 months, 6 through 11 months, 1 through 6 years, and 7 through 10 years were approximately 160, 40, 22, and 30 per 100,000 populations, respectively (196). In 1994 to 1998, _13,800 children less than 2 years old were hospitalized as result of pertussis, whereas in 1999 to 2003, the number of hospitalizations was_17,000 for the same age group (197). In 2003, 19% of total reported pertussis cases (n _ 11,647) occurred in infants aged less than 1 year (198). In 2010, 25 deaths were reported among infants aged less than 6 months (199). In the United States, from 2012 to 2013, 12 pertussis-associated deaths were reported in infants under 3 months of age, and one child died among children aged 1 through 4 years old (200). From 2013 to 2014, seven deaths in infants under 3 months old and one fatality in children 1 through 4 years old were reported (196). Pertussis outbreaks have occurred in several states and in all regions of the United States (201–206). In Ohio, from 2009 through 2010, 2,958 cases were reported (205). Additionally, from May 2010 through May 2011, a mixed pertussis and pertussis-like illness outbreak produced 918 cases in Franklin County, Ohio (34). In 2012, Minnesota experienced a large pertussis epidemic in which 4,144 cases were reported (206). Nationwide, during 2012, the total number of reported pertussis cases in all age groups exceeded 48,000, including 20 pertussis-related deaths that occurred primarily in infants aged less than 3 months (207). From 2012 through 2014, 6,231 cases were reported from Washington State. In 2012 alone, a majority (31 of 39) of Washington State counties were affected. In the same year (2012), there were 4,918 total cases (including both confirmed and probable cases), with an overall incidence of 11/100,000 residents (203, 208). During this outbreak, 95 infants were diagnosed with pertussis (incidence, 107/ 100,000), including 35 children who required hospitalization (208).

## 3.4.3 BURDEN OF PERTUSSIS IN ADOLESCENTS AND ADULTS

Pertussis among adolescents and adults has been reported with increasing frequency during the last 2 to 3 decades (188, 190, 215–233). Population-based studies between 1991 and 1999 estimated an incidence of pertussis in adults of 133 to 507 per 100,000 person- years (167, 171, 234–237), which equates to more than one million cases of pertussis among adults in North America annually (167). In 2013, the nationwide incidences of pertussis among persons 11 to 19 years old and 20 years or older were approximately 28 and 21 per 100,000, respectively (200). In the 2014 pertussis outbreak in California, most reported cases were among adolescents aged 9 to 16 years, and whites were more affected than other racial/ethnic groups (201). The observed increase in reported cases among adolescents and adults has been attributed, in part, to waning immunity that occurs several years after primary childhood immunization (216, 239–246). Such waning immunity likely plays an important role in pertussis transmission among household contacts (218, 247–253).

## 3.4.4 TRANSMISSION DYNAMICS OF PERTUSSIS

Pertussis is highly contagious and can spread rapidly from person to- person through contact with airborne droplets. The human nasopharynx can be densely colonized with both commensal bacteria and pathogens, including B. pertussis. Infected individuals aerosolize pertussis-containing droplets by coughing or sneezing (260). Pertussis is considered far more contagious than polio, smallpox, rubella, mumps, and diphtheria (262, 263). Studies showed that one infected person can transmit *Bordetella pertussis*to as many as 12 to 17 other susceptible individuals, (261–266).

## 3.5 IMPACT OF PERTUSSIS

B.pertussis infection can lead to severe disease in adults, resulting in lost work time, clinic or emergency department visits, or hospitalization (226, 238, 272–275). In patients infected with B. pertussis, the incubation period usually lasts 7 to 10 days, but incubation periods as long as 4 weeks have been observed (277). Although pertussis most often presents clinically as whooping cough, the range of signs and symptoms at presentation can vary from the youngest infants to adolescents (Table 3). Infants and children manifest a range of symptoms from asymptomatic or mild upper respiratory tract disease to severe, persistent, and progressive coughing that continues for weeks or months. The classic symptom of pertussis, from which the original name "whooping cough" is derived, consists of violent and rapid coughing with rapid expulsion of air from the lungs, in which the patient is then forced to inhale with a loud "whooping" sound.

Table 1: Clinical manifestations of pertussis among infants, children, adolescents, and adults, 1988 to 2002

| Clinical sign (references) | Frequency (%) i | |
|---|---|---|
| | Infants | Adolescents |
| Coughing paroxysms (167, 219, 226, 234, 273) | 89–93 | 70–99 |
| Inspiratory whoops (167, 219, 224,226, 234, 273, 289, 659) | 69-92 | 8-82 |
| Nocturnal cough (219, 224, 226,232, 660) | 41 | 61-87 |
| Posttussive vomiting (167, 219, 224, 226, 232, 234, 273, 289, 659 | 48-60 | 17-65 |

| No or low-grade fever (234, 659) | 87-96 | 13 |
|---|---|---|
| Coryza (234) | NA | 58 |
| Pharyngitis (234) | NA | 31 |

aAges 6 days to 9 years.

b NA, data not available.

In infants and young children, the clinical course of pertussis progresses through three consecutive stages after infection and incubation: the catarrhal, paroxysmal, and convalescent stages. Each stage lasts approximately 1 to 3 weeks, and the patients typically do not fully recover for 2 to 3 months (155, 272, 278, and 279). In the first stage, the catarrhal stage, infants and children often present with normal body temperature or low-grade fever, malaise, sore throat, nasal congestion, rhinorrhea, lacrimation, sneezing, and mild progressive dry cough. Although coryza, pharyngitis, and nocturnal cough paroxysms are commonly reported, there are limited systematically collected data for these signs. In the catarrhal stage, the diagnosis of pertussis is frequently overlooked by clinicians because these signs and symptoms mimic those in other viral infections associated with rhinoviruses, corona viruses, and influenza viruses and perhaps because they expect the vaccinated child to be protected from pertussis infection (280, 281). At this stage of illness, parents frequently bring children to ambulatory care clinics and emergency departments. In these outpatient settings, clinicians need to maintain a high index of suspicion for pertussis in order to provide appropriate referrals to nearby health facilities that are equipped to deliver emergency supportive care and confirmatory diagnostic testing for pertussis. Delays in diagnosis and treatment of pertussis facilitate its transmission to household contacts, friends, schoolmates, and family members (145, 233, 282).

In the second stage of illness, the paroxysmal stage, patients experience bouts of intense and violent coughing (5 to 10 coughs/ paroxysms) that last several minutes and are associated with cyanosis, eye proptosis, tongue protrusion, salivation, thick oral mucus production, lacrimation, and engorgement of neck veins (163). The classic sign of pertussis, the inspiratory whoops, manifests at this stage (283). Coughing paroxysms may result from the effects of toxin or from the hardening of mucus that becomes difficult to dislodge from the trachea, bronchi, or bronchioles. Paroxysms can be triggered by stimuli such as crying, laughing, and eating (284). Such paroxysms often occur at night and increase in frequency during the first 1 to 2 weeks of this stage through weeks 2 to 3, with a gradual decline thereafter. In the paroxysmal stage, patients might also experience vomiting (posttussive vomiting), fatigue, and respiratory exhaustion.

In the third stage, convalescence, coughing paroxysms recede in frequency, duration, and severity. However, a mild, chronic, nonparoxysmal cough can last up to 6 weeks. In children who have had the classic type of pertussis, cough paroxysm patterns can recur if the child contracts another viral infection (145, 272, and 278). By this stage, patients will have already received appropriate antibiotic and supportive therapy. Adolescents and adults present with signs and symptoms similar to those in infants and children. In general, however, most adolescents and adults have symptoms that are milder than those of infants and children are; consequently, pertussis in adolescents and adults can escape detection by clinicians (233, 285–287). Although classic pertussis presentation can still occur in many patients, pertussis without the classic paroxysms is the cause of up to one-third of illnesses with prolonged cough in this age group (219, 288). Therefore, pertussis should be highly suspected as a cause of cough that persists for more than 3 weeks, regardless of whether it is paroxysmal (288). In adolescents and adults, cough duration ranges from 3 to 8 weeks (167, 217, 219, 232, 273, 289).

Studies suggested that the clinical presentation of pertussis is influenced by age, gender, infecting species (e.g., *Bordetellapertussis*versusB. parapertussis), infectious dose, and time from last pertussis vaccination (144, 145, 218, 290). Symptomatic reinfections are common in adolescents and adults (273, 291). In a pertussis vaccine efficacy trial of 246 adults conducted between 1991 and 1994, 64 subjects of whom 26% had a history of pertussis infection (234). In older adults, the classic whooping cough can be dramatic, as demonstrated by a recent case study of pertussis in a hospitalized adult (292). Also, in older adults, the clinical presentation of pertussis migh11.t be influenced by preexisting immunity to *Bordetella pertussis*as a result of previous exposure or immunization. Adults who had been recently immunized or had a previous pertussis infection tended to have less dramatic presentation, particularly those lacking comorbid medical conditions (144, 145, 218, 290).

## 3.6 POSTEXPOSURE PROPHYLAXIS AND THERAPEUTICS

The selection of antimicrobial agent should be driven based on the following considerations: age of the patient, drug-related adverse events or interactions, tolerability, medication regimen adherence, and cost. A limited number of antibiotic agents are available for pertussis management, including PEP in individuals who come in contact with clinical cases of pertussis. (278, 332–335). The decision to administer PEP isbased on many factors, including the severity of disease, durationand burden of exposure, and immune competence of the exposedcontact (278). Antimicrobial agents are recommended to clear the nasopharynxof *Bordetella pertussis*and to prevent the spread of the infection(332, 336, 337). It was estimated that 80% to 90% of patients withuntreated pertussis will clear *Bordetella pertussis*from the nasopharynxwithin 3 to 4 weeks after the onset of cough (338). However, infantswith pertussis who were not treated or vaccinated showedpositive culture for more than 6 weeks (339). Macrolide antibiotics (e.g., erythromycin, clarithromycin, orazithromycin) have been effective and constitute the mainstay oftreatment for patients with pertussis as well as for PEP (278). Among the three most widely prescribed macrolides, azithromycinis the only recommended antimicrobial for neonates (_1month old) (278). For children and adults, azithromycin, clarithromycin, orerythromycin may be used (278, 342).

### 3.6.1 Nonmacrolide Treatments

Trimethoprim-sulfamethoxazole (also known as co-trimoxazole) is used as an alternative to macrolides but should be used only in children older than 1 month and in adults when macrolides are not well tolerated (278). Because of the potential risk for kernicterus among infants, co-trimoxazole should not be administered to pregnant women, nursing mothers, or infants aged less than 2 months (278).

## 3.7 IMMUNITY TO PERTUSSIS

Immunity to pertussis, acquired either from natural infection or through vaccination, is not lifelong. It has been estimated that natural pertussis infection yields 3.5 to 30 years of protection (383–386); the estimated protection obtained from the whole-cell pertussis vaccine is 5 to 14 years (387–393), and that from the acellular vaccine is 4 to 7 years (241, 390, 394–397). As a result of waninimmunity over time, adolescents and adults are susceptible to infection with B. pertussis. The severity of their disease appears to be strongly linked to the time since previous vaccination or illness due to *Bordetella pertussis*(215, 398).

## 3.8 VACCINES AND IMMUNIZATIONS

### 3.8.1 DTP and DTaP Vaccines for Infants and Young Children

In 1976, the number of pertussis cases reported to the U.S. CDC reached its nadir at approximately 1,000 (144, 271, 474–476). In the United States, the whole-cell pertussis vaccine has been administered to children in combination with diphtheria and tetanus toxoids. Whole-cell pertussis vaccines, consisting of suspensions of inactivated B. pertussis, elicit humoral immunity to pertussis following intramuscular injection (477). Based on that concept, the first evidence of DTP vaccine efficacy was obtained from a clinical trialconducted during the 1929 pertussis outbreak in the Faroe Islands of Denmark (478, 479). In the 1930s, many steps were taken to improve DTP vaccines, including increasing the number of inactivated *Bordetella pertussis*bacteria in the vaccine, standardizing the methods used to grow and kill the bacteria, and using fresh, rapidly growing phase one bacteria as the inoculum (62, 480). As a result, a variety of DTP vaccines were produced in the United States, which varied in their methods of production and generated different levels of antibody response (480, 481). Previous observational studies and clinical trials showed 70% to 90% efficacy of DTP vaccines to prevent serious pertussis disease (158, 482–484). To enhance the immunogenicity of the vaccine and reduce its adverse effects, vaccine was adsorbed onto an aluminum salt(284). In 1970s, confidence in DTP vaccines began to decline in several countries after reports of local and systemic reactions surfaced in several locations (Table 6). In addition to reports of local skin reactions at the injection site, other less common but more serious systemic adverse events were linked to DTP, including neurological diseases such as encephalopathy, infantile spasms, and sudden infant death syndrome (485–487). Moreover, growing medical and public anxiety coupled with a heightened molecular structural knowledge of *Bordetella pertussis*led to production of less reactogenic acellular pertussis vaccines (284). In Japan, Sato et al. designed the first purified-component DTaP vaccine (488). The initial acellular vaccines (Takeda-type vaccines) consisted predominantly of FHA, small amounts of inactivated PT, and, in some cases, fimbrial proteins and PRN. These constructs were followed by development of other acellular (Biken-type) vaccines containing equal amounts of PT and FHA. Newer DTaP vaccines contained purified immunogenic antigens and excluded LPS, which was present in the DTP vaccines (473, 489–493). In addition, the new-generation DTaP vaccines underwent rigorous testing for potential toxicity and potency in mice, while testing for potential adverse events and antibody response was done in children. The results of safety testing were reassuring and revealed that the efficacy of DTaP vaccines exceeded that of whole-cell DTP vaccines. Larger effectiveness trials and pertussis surveillance studies followed and proved that DTaP vaccines were effective and safe (284). The incidence rates of pertussis for the years 2013 and 2014 were approximately 151, 40, 22, 30, 25, and 2 per 100,000 persons for the age groups less than 6 months, 6 to 11 months, 1 to 6 years, 7 to 10 years, 11 to 19 years, and _20 years, respectively (500). In the 2010 EUVAC pertussis surveillance report, the incidence rates of pertussis across Europe were 15, 4, 5, 13, 10, and 2 cases per 100,000 persons for the age groups less than 1 year, 1 to 4 years, 5 to 9 years, 10 to 14 years, 15 to 19 years, and _20 years of age, respectively (501). The prevention of pertussis centers on the provision of pertussis vaccines in routine childhood immunization programs. These programs vary across countries where licensed pertussis vaccines have been administered to infants, children, and adults. In the United States, and based on the guidelines of the Advisory Committee on Immunization Practices (ACIP), the childhood immunization schedule for DTaP vaccine consists of five doses for children less than 7 years of age. These five doses are given at 2, 4, 6, and 15 to 18 months of age, and one booster dose is given at 4 to 6 years of age (515, 516). Although DTaP vaccines became widely used in many countries, including the United States, Canada, and Australia, in some Asian and many

European countries, DTP vaccines are still the mainstay of pertussis prevention (182, 432, 517–519). In the United States, despite great success of public health programs and availability of vaccines for disadvantaged children through the federally funded Vaccines for Children Program, many children in medically underserved areas as well as in minority groups remain partially immunized or nonimmunized (520). Recent (2015) data from Detroit, MI, show that only 40% of children have completed the primary vaccination series and suggest that rates of under immunization may exceed 50% in some populations (Michigan Care Improvement Registry, unpublished data). Such under immunization suggests the need for improved local-, state-, and national-level immunization strategies to reach the Healthy People 2020 goals of 95% vaccine coverage for several pediatric vaccines (521).

### 3.8.2 DIAGNOSIS

In suspected pertussis outbreaks, control measures begin by first confirming pertussis among affected individuals. To confirm the illness, clinical specimens (e.g., nasopharyngeal swabs) are collected and tested. According to the U.S. CDC, diagnosis of pertussis in outbreak situations is best done by culture (333). Given the potential for false-positive results associated with PCR, the U.S. CDC advises exercising caution in using PCR during outbreak investigations. Pulsed-field gel electrophoresis (PFGE) is currently the most widely used method to track transmission patterns in an outbreak and characterize *Bordetella pertussis*strains (462). Newer PFGE methods offer the potential for improved standardization and comparison of *Bordetella pertussis*strains detected in different laboratories (333, 462). Recently, a new strain-typing technique called single nucleotide primer extension (SNPeX) was developed and showed promise as a flexible and time-efficient way to study outbreaks of *Bordetella pertussis*and other pathogens (464). SNPeX analyzes fluorescently labeled DNA fragments with high-throughput capacity, a high degree of discrimination, and adaptability for detecting strains that may evolve and vary genetically within outbreaks or from one outbreak to another. (333).

### 3.8.3 TYPES OF VACCINES

Currently, both whole-cell and acellular pertussis vaccines are distributed by manufacturers in Belgium, Bulgaria, France, India, Indonesia, Italy, and South Korea. Whole-cell vaccines are available in combination with conjugate *Haemophilusinfluenzae*type B vaccine, enhanced inactivated poliovirus vaccine, or hepatitis B virus vaccine (284). Since 1996, in the United States, only acellular pertussis-containing vaccines are shown in the recommended immunization schedule.

There are five U.S. Food and Drug Administration- licensed DTaP vaccines for infants and young children, and they vary in the amount and number of antigens in the vaccine. In addition to diphtheria and tetanus toxoids, the vaccines also contain other pertussis components as follows. Certiva (Baxter Laboratories) is a monocomponent vaccine that contains only PT antigen. Tripedia (Sanofi Pasteur) is a dual-component vaccine containing PT and FHA, while Infanrix (GlaxoSmithKline) is a triple-component vaccine containing PT, FHA, and PRN. In the United States, the combination of Infanrix, hepatitis B vaccine, and inactivated poliovirus vaccine is marketed as Pediarix (Glaxo- SmithKline). Pediarix is supplied in single-dose, thimerosal-free vials or prefilled syringes and is licensed for a three-dose primary series in infants born to mothers without hepatitis B surface antigen. Acel-Immune (no longer manufactured) and Daptacel (Sanofi Pasteur) are four-component vaccines that contain PT, FHA, PRN, and FIM2 (Acel-Immune) or PT, FHA, PRN, and FIM2, 3 (Daptacel) (163, 284).

Tdap vaccines (under the brand names Adacel and Boostrix) are licensed in the United States for immunization of adolescents and adults. Adacel (Sanofi Pasteur) is a five-component acellular pertussis vaccine. Adacel is licensed for use in the United States in persons 11 to 64 years old and is supplied in thimerosal-free, single- dose vials. Boostrix (GlaxoSmithKline) is a three-component acellular pertussis vaccine. In the United States, Boostrix is licensed for use in persons 10 years of age and older (284).

## 3.9 PROTEIN PURIFICATION

### 3.9.1 AIM OF PROTEIN PURIFICATION

The main aim of protein purification is to retain larger amount of proteins with the fewest contaminants. Proteins are isolated from their sources such as tissue, or model organisms like bacteria, fungi, yeast or mammalian cells in culture; based on the differences in their physical properties.

Usually a protein purification protocol contains one or more chromatographic steps. The basic procedure in chromatography is to flow the solution containing the protein through a column packed with various materials. Different proteins interact differently with the column material, and can thus be separated by the time required to pass the column, or the conditions required to elute the protein from the column. Usually proteins are detected as they are coming off the column by their absorbance at 280 nm.

### 3.9.2 TYPES OF CHROMATOGRAPHIC SYSTEM

Many different chromatographic methods exist:

## SIZE EXLUSION:

- ➢ It is also called as gel permeation chromatography
- ➢ Size exclusion chromatography can be used to separate protein in solution or denaturing conditions by using porous gels
- ➢ he principle is that smaller molecules have to traverse a larger volume in a porous matrix
- ➢ Proteins of a certain range in size will require a variable volume of eluent (solvent) before being collected at the other end of the column of gel

## BASED ON CHARGE:

### ❖ HIC (HYDROPHOBIC INTERACTION CHROMATOGRAPHY)

- ➢ HIC media is amphiphilic, with both hydrophobic and hydrophilic regions, allowing forseparation of proteins based on their surface hydrophobicity
- ➢ Target proteins and their product aggregate species tend to have different hydrophobic properties and removing them via HIC further purifies the protein of interest

## ION EXCHANGE CHROMATOGRAPHY

- ➢ Ion exchange chromatography separates compounds according to the nature an degree of their ionic charge
- ➢ The column to be used is selected according to its type and strength of charge
- ➢ Anion exchange resins have a positive charge and are used to retain and separate negatively charged compounds (anions), while Cation exchange resins have a negative charge and are used to separate positively charged molecules (cations)

## HPLC:

High performance liquid chromatography or high pressure liquid chromatography is a form of chromatography applying high pressure to drive the solutes through the column faster. This means that the diffusion is limited and the resolution is improved. The most common form is "reversed phase" HPLC, where the column material is hydrophobic. The proteins are eluted by a gradient of increasing amounts of an organic solvent, such as acetonitrile. The proteins elute according to their hydrophobicity. After purification by HPLC the protein is in a solution that only contains volatile compounds, and can easily be lyophilized.HPLC purification frequently results in denaturation of the purified proteins and is thus not applicable to proteins that do not spontaneously refold.

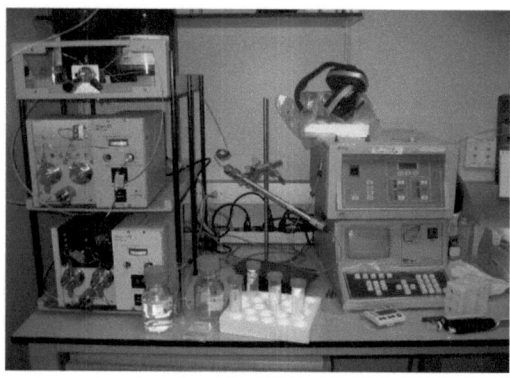

Figure 1: : High performance liquid chromatography

# 4. MATERIALS AND METHODS

- Tangential flow filtration system
- Chromatographic system
- Dialysis membrane
- Buffers
- Centrifuge system
- Magnetic stirrer
- Milli-Q system
- Water bath
- Laminar air flow hood
- Pipettes
- Weighing balance
- pH and conductivity meter
- Glass wares
- 0.2 micron filters
- Falcon tubes

CHEMICALS REQUIRED:

- disodium hydrogen phosphate
- formaldehyde,
- glacial acetic acid,
- glutaraldehyde,
- glycine,
- hydrochloric acid,
- monopotassium orthophosphate,
- N-acetyl tryptophan,
- ortho phosphoric acid,
- sodium acetate,
- sodium bi carbonate,
- sodium carbonate,

- Sodium chloride,
- sodium dihydrogen phosphate,
- sodium hydroxide,
- sulphuric acid,
- Tween-20
- urea,

## 4.1TANGENTIAL FLOW FILTRATION

Tangential flow filtration system:

It is also called as cross-flow filtration. In this the feed stream passes parallel to the membrane face as one portion passes the membrane (permeate) while the remaining (retentate) is recirculated back to the feed reservoir. The main applications of tangential flow filtration are concentration and diafiltration.

Concentration:

Concentration is a simple process that involves removing fluid from a solution while retaining the solute molecules. The concentration of the solute increases in direct proportion to the decrease in solution volume, i.e. halving the volume effectively doubles the concentration

Diafiltration:

Diafiltration is the fractionation process that washes smaller molecules through a membrane and leaves larger molecules in the retentate without ultimately changing concentration. It can be used to remove salts or exchange buffers.

Sample processing (concentration):

- ➢ Clean containers and tubing connections are arranged
- ➢ Feed container was filled with the sample to be concentrated
- ➢ Pump set at the required crossflow rate was turned on
- ➢ The sample was filtered until the desired concentration or volume is obtained
- ➢ The pump was turned off and the feed tubing from the feed container was removed

- ➤ The pump was turned on and the retentate and upstream fluid was collected in the feed container
- ➤ Pump was turned off and the feed tubing was removed

Product recovery:

- ➤ Feed tubing was placed in the feed container
- ➤ The permeate tubing was removed from the permeate port and replaced with cap
- ➤ The retentate tubing was removed from retentate port and the other end was kept in the feed container
- ➤ End of the retentate tube was held higher than the feed container in order to drain the sample out
- ➤ 5 ml of buffer filled in 25 ml syringe was attached to the retentate port
- ➤ Slowly buffer was pushed into the device and syringe was disconnected
- ➤ Syringe was filled with air and reconnected to the retentate port to push the air into the device
- ➤ Remaining sample in the feed tubing was recovered by removing the tubing from the device and the sample was drained into the feed container

## 4.2 COLUMN CHROMATOGRAPHIC SYSTEM

Column chromatography is commonly used to purify compounds made in the lab. The process of washing a compound through a column using a solvent is known as elution. The solvent is sometimes known as eluent.

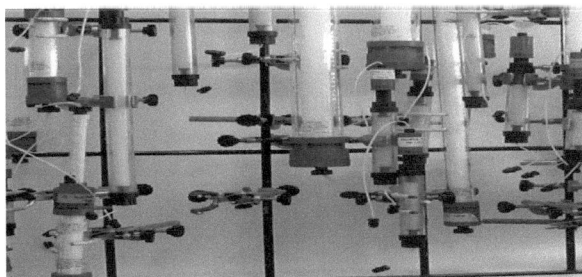

Figure 2:Column chromatographic system

PACKING OF COLUMN:

Column is packed in different ways depending on column type and equipment used. Column packing is of two types:

1. Pressure/ Flow packing (column with adapter)
2. Suction packing(in large column with fixed bed height)

SLURRY PREPARATION

> Packing solution (slurry) is either with water or running buffer

> Determine desired packed bed volume using the formula below:

$$\text{Column volume (CV)} = \left(\frac{\pi d^2}{4}\right) * l$$

Where,

$l$ = desired bed height

$\frac{\pi d^2}{4}$=cross-sectional area of column

> Gently shake the resin bottle to make an even slurry
> Measure the required volume of resin slurry i.e., *1.2\*desired packed resin volume* using a measuring cylinder
> Suspend resin by shaking in the measuring cylinder and pour to a funnel
> Wash 5 times with 2 CVs
> Gently stir with spatula between additions and shift it to beaker
> Dilute resin suspension with packing solution to form 50-70% slurry
> Stir gently with glass rod to make homogenous suspension (never use magnetic stirrer for mixing)

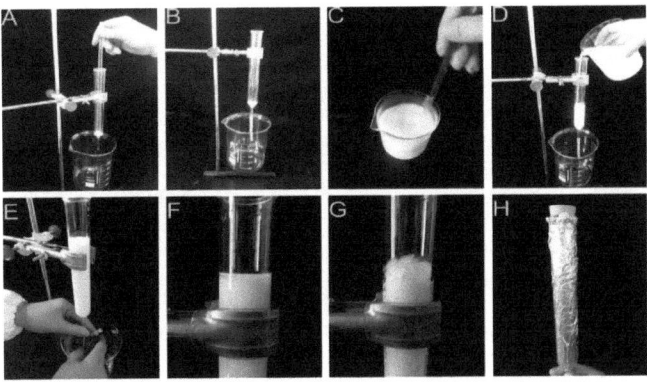

Figure 3:Slurry preparation and column packing

COLUMN PACKING

We usually use pressure flow packing. Pressure packing columns are packed by conventional pressure packing by pumping the packing solution through the chromatographic bed at constant flow velocity.

STEPS

1. Pour some water into the column, make sure that no air is trapped under the bottom of the net. Leave 2cm of liquid in column.
2. Prepare 50-70% resin slurry. Pour slurry into the column. Insert the adapter and lower it into the surface of slurry, make sure no air is trapped below the adapter.
3. Seal the adapter O-ring and lower the adapter a little into the slurry enough to fill the adapter inlet with packing solution.
4. Connect the pump and pressure meter and start packing the recommended flow rate. Keep the flow rate constant during packing and check the pressure at column inlet.
5. When the resin has settled, mark the bed height on the column tube, close the bottom valve and stop the pump. The bed starts rising in the column. Loosen the O-ring and lower the adapter to about 0.5-1.0cm from the resin surface.
6. Seal the O-ring, start the pump and continue packing at the recommended packing flow rate. Repeat steps 5 and 6 until there is a maximum of 1cm between resin surface and adapter when resin has stabilized.
7. Close the bottom valve, stop the pump, disconnect the column inlet and push the adapter down approximately 3mm below the mark on the column tube without loosening the adapter O-ring.

8. The packing solution will flush the adapter inlet. Remove any trapped air by pumping liquid from the bottom.

## Steps involved during the manual run of chromatographic system

Parameters to be set in the system:

- System flow
- Pre-column pressure
- Sample flow
- pH valve
- column position
- alarm air sensors
- alarm system pressure

Before loading the sample:

- ➢ Connect the packed column to the system and switch it on
- ➢ Set the parameters required for wash and equilibration of the column
- ➢ Initially 3-4 CVs of water wash was done to the column
- ➢ Then for removing impurities wash with 0.5N NaOH for 1-2 CVs and give water wash for 2-3 CVs
- ➢ Pass regeneration buffer (NaCl) of 2-3 CVs for resin activation and again water wash for 2-3 CVs
- ➢ For column equilibration pass the required buffer for 5-6 CVs

After loading the sample:

- ➢ After equilibration load the sample ; the load flow rate should be lower than the flow rate during equilibration or efficient protein binding
- ➢ Post load wash was done with the same buffer used for equilibration for 2-3 CVs
- ➢ Finally elution of proteins were done with the help of elution buffer based on the U.V and the peak formed
- ➢ After elution ,water and NaOH wash was done for 2-3 CVs for CIP(Cleaning-in-place)

## 4.3 DIALYSIS

It is a separation technique that facilitates the removal of small, unwanted compounds from macromolecules in solution by selective and passive diffusion through a semi-permeable membrane. It is used to perform purification or buffer exchange for samples containing macro molecules. A dialysis membrane is a semi-permeable film (usually a sheet of regenerated cellulose) containing various sized pores. A sample and a buffer solution (called the dialysate, usually 200-300 times the volume of the sample) are placed on opposite sides of the membrane. Sample molecule that are larger than the membrane-pores are retained on the sample side of the membrane, but small molecules and buffer salts pass freely through the membrane, reducing the concentration of those molecules in the sample. Changing the dialysate buffer removes the small molecules that are no longer in the sample and allows more contaminants to diffuse into the dialysate. In this way the concentration of small contaminants with in the sample can be decrease to negligible levels.

Materials:

- Protein sample
- Dialysate buffer
- Dialysis membrane
- Container to hold the buffer

Processing of dialysis membrane:

➤ Tube was washed with running water for 3-4 hrs to remove glycerol
➤ Tubing is treated with 0.3% sodium sulfide solution at 80°C for 1min to remove sulfate salts
➤ Washed with hot water(60°C) for 2min,followed by acidification with 0.2% sulphuric acid solution and rinsed with hot water to remove the acid

Procedure:

✓ Prepared the membrane according to instructions
✓ Loaded the sample into dialysis tubing and dialyzed for 2hrs
✓ Changed the dialysis buffer and dialyzed for another 2 hrs
✓ Changed the dialysis buffer and dialyzed overnight at 4°C

# 5. PROCEDURE

Acellular pertussis vaccine requires fermentation, isolation and purification of antigenic components i.e. pertussis toxoid (PT), filamentous hemagglutinin (FHA), pertactin (69kD protein), fimbriae and The number of doses per fermentation batch of acellular pertussis vaccine is usually 20-25 times lower than whole cell pertussis vaccine.

1. A fermentation batch was harvested for the separation of supernatant and pellet
2. This supernatant was used for the extraction of PT and FHA; while the pellet was used to extract PRN.

## 5.1 PROCESS FOR PT AND FHA PURIFICATION:

➤ The supernatant from the harvest was concentrated using Tangential Flow Filtration system.

➤ During the first stage of tangential flow filtration UF permeate and UF retentate were obtained.

➤ The UF retentate acquired was concentrated with phosphate buffer of required composition to procure DF retentate

➤ Parallelly chromatographic system set up was done i.e., slurry preparation, column packing and the column was washed and equilibrated with the corresponding buffers before the sample(DF retentate) was loaded

➤ To the DF retentate 10% of tween-20 was added to prevent the aggregation

➤ This DF retentate(load) was loaded onto anion exchange column chromatographic

➤ The chromatographic system was manually run and the proteins PT and FHA were eluted at different salt concentrations (PT was eluted first with the lower salt concentration and FHA at later stage with little higher salt concentration) and were collected separately in different tubes and they were analysed for protein content and SDS-PAGE.

➤ After the analysis of protein content the PT containing samples were pooled together and FHA containing samples were also pooled together respectively in a separate glass bottles.

## 5.2 PROCESS FOR PRN PURIFICATION:

➤ The pellet from the harvest was agitated with $1^{st}$ extraction buffer using impeller till it was homogenized

➤ This homogenized mixture was centrifuged 7000rpm almost for an hour

> The supernatant was collected and the pellet settled was mixed with 2nd extraction buffer and was kept in water bath at 60°C for 90 min for increasing cell wall permeability
> This was then centrifuged and the supernatant was collected
> Both the supernatants were mixed together and the mixture was loaded into the chromatographic system
> The Multi Modal ion exchange chromatographic system was run and the PRN protein was eluted and sent for analysis
> PRN containing samples were pooled together

3. All the pooled samples of PT, FHA and PRN were concentrated separately using tangential flow filtration and the DF retentate of the three protein samples were collected separately
4. All the collected samples were finally filtered with 0.22µm filter and the proteins were stored at 2-8°C until use.
5. As PT protein has the toxic property, before preparation of acellular pertussis vaccine, PT was detoxified with detoxifying agents.
6. Detoxification was done using detoxifying agents followed by formulation
7. The formulated product obtained was pertussis vaccine.
8. Further the vaccine safety and immunogenicity were evaluated in the animal model.

Note: After each and every single step the samples are taken for analysis

# 6. RESULTS

## Purification of Pertussis Toxin (PT) and FHA from *Bordetella pertussis*

The fermentation harvest was clarified by using centrifugation and the pellet and supernatant were collected separately. PT and FHA were purified from the supernatant and PRN from cell pellet.

PT and FHA were purified by the method explained in the procedure section with the help of an anion exchange chromatography metod. In this process PT eluted first and is collected as PT fraction and FHA eluted in the second fraction and is collected as FHA fraction.

Purified PT and FHA meets the purity specifications for preparation of a vaccine component. The SDS-PAGE gel picture of the same is shown in the below picture.

### SD_PAGE profile of PT, FHA and PRN proteins

| Well No. | Sample Description | Protein Load (μg) | 1 | 2 | 3 | 4 | 5 | 6 | 7 | 8 | 9 | 10 |
|---|---|---|---|---|---|---|---|---|---|---|---|---|
| Purified PT, FHA and PRN proteins from *Bordetella pertussis* | | | | | | | | | | | | |
| 1 | Blank | NA | | | | | | | | | | |
| 2 | Purified Pertussis Toxin (PT) | 3.98 | | | | | | | | | | |
| 3 | Purified Pertussis Toxin (FHA) | 2.33 | | | | | | | | | | |
| 4 | Purified Pertussis Toxin (PRN) | 1.80 | | | | | | | | | | |
| 5 | Blank | NA | | | | | | | | | | |
| 6 | Protein Molecular Weght Marker | 15μL | | | | | | | | | | |
| 7 | BSA as Molecular Weght Marker | 0.10 | | | | | | | | | | |
| 8 | BSA as Molecular Weght Marker | 0.20 | | | | | | | | | | |
| 9 | BSA as Molecular Weght Marker | 0.30 | | | | | | | | | | |
| 10 | BSA as Molecular Weght Marker | 0.40 | | | | | | | | | | |
| Mol.Wt. Marker: 250, 150, 100, 75, 50, 37, 25, 20, 15 & 10 kDa (Top to bottom). | | | | | | | | | | | | |

## Purification of Pertactin protein from *Bordetella pertussis*

Pertactin(69k) membrane protein was purified by the method explained in the procedure section with the help of a Multi Modal Ion exchange chromatography method. In this process the bound PRN was eluted with changing the pH of the column mobile phase and the eluted PRN was collected separately and analysed for protein content and SDS_PAGE.

Purified Pertactin(69K) protein meets the purity specifications for preparation of a vaccine component. The SDS-PAGE gel picture of the same is shown in the above picture.

## Process development

Purification of the PT, FHA and PRN were done at a scale of 15L&30L fermentation scale and purification procedure was optimized.

The process of purification of PT, FHA and PRN is optimized to robust and consistent process by evaluating several fermentations runs followed by purification process.

Hence the purification process optimized and developed at a scale of 15Land 30L fermentation scale with consistency and robustness.

## Summary:

In summary the purification of Bordetella pertussis, proteins; PT, FHA and PRN were purified using novel modern chromatography purification process was developed with consistency and robustness. Further the purified vaccine components can be formulated to prepare the acellular pertussis vaccine product. Acellular pertussis vaccine got most importance as the prevailing toxicity with the existing whole cell pertussis vaccine. So the development of novel acellular pertussis vaccine will protect the childrens from the side effects of the existing wP vaccines.

# REFERENCES

1. Melief CJ, van Hall T, Arens R, Ossendorp F, van der Burg SH (September 2015). *"Therapeutic cancer vaccines"*. The Journal of Clinical Investigation. 125 (9): 3401–12. *doi:10.1172/JCI80009. PMC 4588240. PMID 26214521.*

2. Bol KF, Aarntzen EH, Pots JM, OldeNordkamp MA, van de Rakt MW, Scharenborg NM, de Boer AJ, van Oorschot TG, Croockewit SA, Blokx WA, Oyen WJ, Boerman OC, Mus RD, van Rossum MM, van der Graaf CA, Punt CJ, Adema GJ, Figdor CG, de Vries IJ, Schreibelt G (March 2016). "Prophylactic vaccines are potent activators of monocyte-derived dendritic cells and drive effective anti-tumor responses in melanoma patients at the cost of toxicity". Cancer Immunology, Immunotherapy. 65 (3): 327–39. doi:10.1007/s00262-016-1796-7. PMC 4779136. PMID 26861670.

3. Brotherton J (2015). "HPV prophylactic vaccines: lessons learned from 10 years experience". Future Virology. 10 (8): 999–1009. doi:10.2217/fvl.15.60.

4. Frazer IH (May 2014). "Development and implementation of papillomavirus prophylactic vaccines". Journal of Immunology. 192(9): 4007–11. doi:10.4049/jimmunol.1490012. PMID 24748633.

5. United States Centers for Disease Control and Prevention (2011). A CDC framework for preventing infectious diseases.Archived 2017-08-29 at the Wayback Machine Accessed 11 September 2012. "Vaccines are our most effective and cost-saving tools for disease prevention, preventing untold suffering and saving tens of thousands of lives and billions of dollars in healthcare costs each year."

6. Hewlett, Erik L.; Damron, F. Heath; Wong, Ting; Fernandez, Julieta; Sisti, Federico; Zacca, Federico; Gonyar, Laura A.; Hoffman, Casandra L. (2019-06-25). "Bordetella pertussis Can Be Motile and Express Flagellum-Like Structures". mBio. 10 (3): e00787–19. doi:10.1128/mBio.00787-19. ISSN 2150-7511. PMC 6520453. PMID 31088927.https://en.wikipedia.org/wiki/Protein_purification

7. Poolman JT, Hallander HO (February 2007). "Acellular pertussis vaccines and the role of pertactin and fimbriae". Expert Rev Vaccines. 6 (1): 47–56. doi:10.1586/14760584.6.1.47. PMID 17280478.

8. Emsley P, Charles IG, Fairweather NF, Isaacs NW (May 1996). "Structure of Bordetella pertussis virulence factor P.69 pertactin". Nature. 381 (6577): 90–2. doi:10.1038/381090a0. PMID 8609998.

9. Jump up to:[a] [b] [c] [d] Inatsuka CS, Xu Q, Vujkovic-Cvijin I, Wong S, Stibitz S, Miller JF, Cotter PA (July 2010). "Pertactin is required for Bordetella species to resist neutrophil-mediated clearance". Infection and Immunity. 78 (7): 2901– doi:10.1128/IAI.00188 PMC 2897405. PMID 20421378.

10. **Nobelprize.org.** 1919.The Nobel Prize in Physiology or Medicine1919-Jules Bordet.http://www.nobelprize.org/nobel_prizes/medicine/laureates/1919/index.html. Accessed 3 October 2015.

11. **Clinical and Laboratory Standards Institute.**2008. Interpretive criteriafor identification of bacteria and fungi by DNA target sequencing; approvedguideline. Clinical and Laboratory Standards Institute, Wayne,PA.http://www.clsi.org/standards/. Accessed 21 March 2015.

12. **McGowan KL, Garcia LS.**2007. Bordetella cultures, p 1– *In* Garcia LS(Ed), Clinical microbiology procedures handbook, 3rd ed. ASM Press, Washington DC

13. **Leber AL.** 2014. Pertussis: relevant species and diagnostic update.ClinLab Med **34**:237–255. http://dx.doi.org/10.1016/j.cll.2014.02.003.

14. **Todar K.** 2012. Bordetella pertussis and whooping cough.*In* Todar'sonline textbook of bacteriology. http://textbookofbacteriology.net/pertussis.html.

15. **Gllllgan PH, Fisher MC.** 1984. Importance of culture in laboratory Diagnosis of Bordetella pertussis infections. J Clin Microbial**20**:891–893.

16. **Hoppe JE, Schlagenhauf M.** 1989. Comparison of three kinds of blood and two incubation atmospheres for cultivation of Bordetella pertussis on charcoal agar. J ClinMicrobiol**27**:2115–2117.

17. **Guthrie JL, Robertson AV, Tang P, Jamieson F, Drews SJ.** 2010. Novel duplex real-time PCR assay detects Bordetellaholmesii in specimens from patients with pertussis-like symptoms in Ontario, Canada. J ClinMicrobiol**48**:1435–1437. http://dx.doi.org/10.1128/JCM.02417-09.

18. **Rodgers L, Martin SW, Cohn A, Budd J, Marcon M, Terranella A, Mandal S, Salamon D, Leber A, Tondella ML, Tatti K, Spicer K, Emanuel A, Koch E, McGlone L, Pawloski L, Lemaile-Williams M, Tucker N, Iyer R, Clark TA, Diorio M.** 2013. Epidemiologic andlaboratory features of a large outbreak of pertussis-like illnesses associated with

cocirculatingBordetellaholmesii and Bordetella pertussis— Ohio, 2010-2011. Clin Infect Dis **56:**322–331. http://dx.doi.org/10.1 /cid/cis888.

19. **Cotter PA, Miller JF.**2001. Bordetella, p 619–674. *In* Groisman EA (ed),Principles of bacterial pathogenesis. Academic Press, New York, NY.

20. **Diavatopoulos DA, Cummings CA, Schouls LM, Brinig MM, RelmanDA, Mooi FR.** 2005. Bordetella pertussis, the causative agent of whoopingcough, evolved from a distinct, human-associated                          lineage                          of B.bronchiseptica.PLoSPathog**1:**e45.http://dx.doi.org/10.1371/journal.ppat0010045.

21. **Mattoo S, Foreman-Wykert AK, Cotter PA, Miller JF.** 2001. Mechanisms of Bordetella pathogenesis. Front Biosci**6:**E168–E186. http://dx.doi.org/10.2741/Mattoo.

22. **Guiso N.** 2009. Bordetella pertussis and pertussis vaccines.Clin InfectDis **49:**1565–1569. http://dx.doi.org/10.1086/644733.

23. **Geisbert TW, Hensley LE, Kagan E, Yu EZ, Geisbert JB, Daddario- DiCaprio K, Fritz EA, Jahrling PB, McClintock K, Phelps JR, Lee AC, Judge A, Jeffs LB, MacLachlan I.** 2006. Postexposure protection ofguinea pigs against a lethal Ebola virus challenge is conferred by RNAinterference. J Infect Dis **193:**1650–1657. http://dx.doi.org/10.1086 /504267.

24. **Locht C, Antoine R, Jacob-Dubuisson F.** 2001. Bordetella pertussis, molecular pathogenesis under                          multiple                          aspects.CurrOpinMicrobiol**4:**82–89. http://dx.doi.org/10.1016/S13695274(00)00169-7.

25. **Morse SI, Morse JH.** 1976. Isolation and properties of the leukocytosisandlymphocytosis-promoting      factor      of      Bordetella      pertussis.J      Exp      Med      **143:**1483–1502. http://dx.doi.org/10.1084/jem.143.6.1483.

26. **Nobelprize.org.** 1919. The Nobel Prize in Physiology or Medicine1919-Jules Bordet. http://www.nobelprize.org/nobel_prizes/medicine/laureates/1919/index.html. Accessed 3 October 2015.

27.**Clinical and Laboratory Standards Institute.** 2008. Interpretive criteriafor identification of bacteria and fungi by DNA target sequencing; approvedguideline. Clinical and Laboratory Standards Institute, Wayne,PA. http://www.clsi.org/standards/. Accessed 21 March 2015.

28.**McGowan KL, Garcia LS.** 2007. Bordetella cultures, p 1– *In* Garcia LS(Ed), Clinical microbiology procedures handbook, 3rd ed. ASM Press, Washington DC

29.**Leber AL.** 2014. Pertussis: relevant species and diagnostic update. ClinLab Med **34:**237–255. http://dx.doi.org/10.1016/j.cll.2014.02.003.

30. **Todar K.** 2012. *Bordetella pertussis* and whooping cough. *In* Todar'sonline textbook of bacteriology. http://textbookofbacteriology.net/pertussis.html.

31. **Gilligan PH, Fisher MC.** 1984. Importance of culture in laboratory Diagnosis of *Bordetella pertussis* infections. J Clin Microbial**20:**891–893.

32. **Hoppe JE, Schlagenhauf M.** 1989. Comparison of three kinds of blood and two incubation atmospheres for cultivation of *Bordetella pertussis*on charcoal agar. J ClinMicrobiol**27:**2115–2117.

33. **Guthrie JL, Robertson AV, Tang P, Jamieson F, Drews SJ.** 2010. Novel duplex real-time PCR assay detects Bordetellaholmesii in specimens from patients with pertussis-like symptoms in Ontario, Canada. J ClinMicrobiol**48:**1435–1437. http://dx.doi.org/10.1128/JCM.02417-09.

34. **Rodgers L, Martin SW, Cohn A, Budd J, Marcon M, Terranella A, Mandal S, Salamon D, Leber A, Tondella ML, Tatti K, Spicer K, Emanuel A, Koch E, McGlone L, Pawloski L, Lemaile-Williams M, Tucker N, Iyer R, Clark TA, Diorio M.** 2013. Epidemiologic and laboratory features of a large outbreak of pertussis-like illnesses associated with cocirculatingBordetellaholmesii and *Bordetella pertussis*— Ohio, 2010-2011. Clin Infect Dis **56:**322–331. http://dx.doi.org/10.1/cid/cis888.

**Cotter PA, Miller JF.** 2001. Bordetella, p 619–674. *In* Groisman EA (ed), Principles of bacterial pathogenesis. Academic Press, New York, NY.

56. **Diavatopoulos DA, Cummings CA, Schouls LM, Brinig MM, Relman DA, Mooi FR.** 2005. *Bordetella pertussis*, the causative agent of whooping cough, evolved from a distinct, human-associated lineage of B. bronchiseptica. PLoSPathog**1:**e45. http://dx.doi.org/10.1371/journal.ppat .0010045.

57. **Mattoo S, Foreman-Wykert AK, Cotter PA, Miller JF.** 2001. Mechanisms of Bordetella pathogenesis. Front Biosci**6:**E168–E186. http://dx.doi.org/10.2741/Mattoo.

58. **Guiso N.** 2009. *Bordetella pertussis* and pertussis vaccines. Clin InfectDis **49:**1565–1569. http://dx.doi.org/10.1086/644733.

59. **Geisbert TW, Hensley LE, Kagan E, Yu EZ, Geisbert JB, Daddario- DiCaprio K, Fritz EA, Jahrling PB, McClintock K, Phelps JR, Lee AC, Judge A, Jeffs LB, MacLachlan I.** 2006. Postexposure protection ofguinea pigs against a lethal Ebola virus challenge is conferred by RNA interference. J Infect Dis **193:**1650–1657. http://dx.doi.org/10.1086 /504267.

60. **Locht C, Antoine R, Jacob-Dubuisson F.** 2001. *Bordetella pertussis*, molecular pathogenesis under multiple aspects. CurrOpinMicrobiol**4:**82–89. http://dx.doi.org/10.1016/S13695274(00)00169-7.

61. **Morse SI, Morse JH.** 1976. Isolation and properties of the leukocytosisandlymphocytosis-promoting factor of *Bordetella pertussis.* J Exp Med **143:**1483–1502. http://dx.doi.org/10.1084/jem.143.6.1483.

62. **Pittman M.** 1984. The concept of pertussis as a toxin-mediated disease. Pediatr Infect Dis **3:**467–486.

63. **Stein PE, Boodhoo A, Armstrong GD, Cockle SA, Klein MH, Read RJ.** 1994. The crystal structure of pertussis toxin. Structure **2:**45–57. http://dx.doi.org/10.1016/S0969-2126(00)00007-1.

64. **Stein PE, Boodhoo A, Armstrong GD, Heerze LD, Cockle SA, Klein MH, Read RJ.** 1994. Structure of a pertussis toxin-sugar complex as amodel for receptor binding. NatStructBiol**1:**591596. http://dx.doi.org/10.1038/nsb0994-591.

65. **Kotob SI, Hausman SZ, Burns DL.** 1995. Localization of the promoter for the ptl genes of *Bordetella pertussis*, which encode proteins essential for secretion of pertussis toxin. Infect Immun**63:**3227–3230.

66. **Confer DL, Eaton JW.** 1982. Phagocyte impotence caused by an invasive bacterial adenylate cyclase. Science **217:**948–950. http://dx.doi.org/10.1126/science.6287574.

67. **Eby JC, Gray MC, Warfel JM, Paddock CD, Jones TF, Day SR, Bowden J, Poulter MD, Donato GM, Merkel TJ, Hewlett EL.** 2013.Quantification of the adenylate cyclase toxin of *Bordetella pertussis* invitro and during respiratory infection. Infect Immun**81:**1390–1398. http://dx.doi.org/10.1128/IAI.00110-13.

68. **El-Azania-El-Idrissi M, Bauche C, Loucka J, Osicka R, Sebo P, LadantD, Leclerc C.** 2003. Interaction of *Bordetella pertussis* adenylate cyclase with CD11b/CD18: role of toxin acylation and identification of the main integrin interaction domain. J BiolChem**278:**38514–38521. http://dx .doi.org/10.1074/jbc.M304387200.

69. **Fiser R, Masin J, Bumba L, Pospisilova E, Fayolle C, Basler M, Sadilkova L, Adkins I, Kamanova J, Cerny J, Konopasek I, Osicka R,Leclerc C, Sebo P.** 2012. Calcium influx rescues adenylatecyclasehemolysinfrom rapid cell membrane removal and enables phagocyte permeabilization by toxin pores. PLoSPathog**8:**e1002580. http://dx.doi.org/10.1371/journal.ppat.1002580.

70. **Glaser P, Danchin A, Ladant D, Barzu O, Ullmann A.** 1988. *Bordetella pertussis* adenylate cyclase: the gene and the protein. Tokai J ExpClinMed **13**(Suppl):239–252.

71. **Glaser P, Elmaoglou-Lazaridou A, Krin E, Ladant D, Barzu O, Danchin A.** 1989. Identification of residues essential for catalysis andbinding of calmodulin in *Bordetella pertussis* adenylate cyclase by sitedirectedmutagenesis. EMBO J **8:**967–972.

72. **Guermonprez P, Khelef N, Blouin E, Rieu P, Ricciardi-Castagnoli P, Guiso N, Ladant D, Leclerc C.** 2001. The adenylate cyclase toxin of*Bordetella pertussis* binds to target cells via the alpha(M)beta(2) integrin(CD11b/CD18). J Exp Med **193:**1035–1044. http://dx.doi.org/10.1084 /jem.193.9.1035.

73. **Hackett M, Guo L, Shabanowitz J, Hunt DF, Hewlett EL.** 1994. Internal lysine palmitoylation in adenylate cyclase toxin from *Bordetella pertussis.* Science **266:**433– 435. http://dx.doi.org/10.1126/science.7939682.

74. **Harvill ET, Cotter PA, Yuk MH, Miller JF.** 1999. Probing the function of Bordetellabronchisepticaadenylate cyclase toxin by manipulating host immunity. Infect Immun**67:**1493–1500.

75. **Henderson MW, Inatsuka CS, Sheets AJ, Williams CL, Benaron DJ, Donato GM, Gray MC, Hewlett EL, Cotter PA.** 2012. Contribution ofBordetella filamentous hemagglutinin and adenylate cyclase toxin tosuppression and evasion of interleukin-17-mediated inflammation. Infect Immun**80:**2061–2075. http://dx.doi.org/10.1128/IAI.00148-12.

76. **Kamanova J, Kofronova O, Masin J,Genth H, Vojtova J, LinhartovaI, Benada O, Just I, Sebo P.** 2008. Adenylate cyclase toxin subvertsphagocyte function by RhoA inhibition and unproductive ruffling. J Immunol**181:**5587–5597. http://dx.doi.org/10.4049/jimmunol.181.8.5587.

77. **Ladant D, Michelson S, Sarfati R, Gilles AM, Predeleanu R, Barzu O.** 1989. Characterization of the calmodulin-binding and of the catalyticdomains of *Bordetella pertussis* adenylate cyclase. J BiolChem**264:**4015–4020.

78. **Paccani SR, Dal Molin F, Benagiano M, Ladant D, D'Elios MM, Montecucco C, Baldari CT.** 2008. Suppression of T-lymphocyteactivation and chemotaxis by the adenylate cyclase toxin of *Bordetella pertussis.* Infect Immun**76:**2822–2832. http://dx.doi.org/10.1128/IAI.00200-08.

# YOUR KNOWLEDGE HAS VALUE

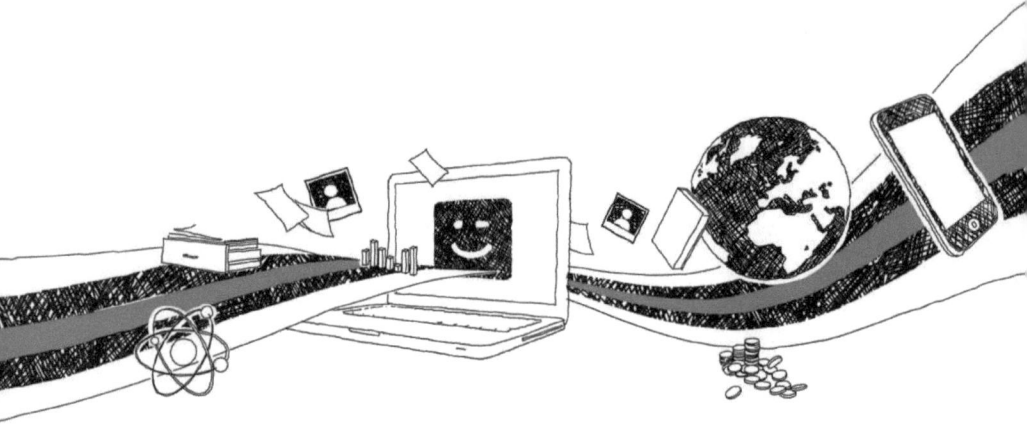

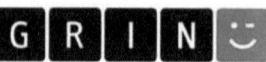